Here It Is

The Cutting Edge of Respite Care

As Envisioned by Isaac Croom Turner, Servant

Foreword by Reverend Floyd Davis

Stay yoked.

Isaac C. Turner, Ph.D

Matt. 11:28,29,30.

Cover Design: SOS Graphics and Designs

ISBN 13: 978-0-9796978-4-5
ISBN 10: 0-9796978-4-0

Published by G Publishing, LLC
P. O. Box 24374
Detroit, MI 48224

Library of Congress Control Number: 2007935621

Printed in the United States of America

DEDICATION

To my dear beloved mother, Dolly Turner Jackson, who was both a Care Giver and Care Recipient role model and follower of the Lamb, and my Uncle Isaac Fluker who carried with himself the ravages of infantile paralysis since age two and to the families and caregivers of the vast numbers of developmentally delayed persons of our society who have captured our attention and hearts and have become our teachers and innovators in yet another needed Christian endeavor. God Bless You and may life minister kindly to you because of your inspiration to read these pages.

A Word of Caution to Those Undertaking This Holy Operandi:

Be sure you observe laws governing the care, touching and handling of children and persons in your care. Above all, be a blessing not a curse.

FOREWORD

Pastor Isaac Turner has written a much needed and often overlooked gift of the body of Christ, the ministry of helps. Although this gift has been termed "Respite Care", the term means the temporary relief of parenting responsibilities on a planned or emergency basis; it is providing spiritual aid helping to extend the abilities of a care provider. If you are a care provider, or persons seeking care for family, you will want to read the lessons and experiences in Pastor Turner's approach.

Care providers take on the task when it involves family and close relationships, not realizing that in the long term experience they will need frequent breaks to be refreshed, restored and revitalized in their attitudes and approach to care giving. Oft times care providers will feel that taking a break or "respite" is shirking their responsibilities or they will feel guilt in the temporary discontinuance of care. The book helps care providers to realize that the break allows them the spiritual opportunity to refocus their care and to think about their own needs while their loved one is under the watchful eye of another. The book shares the care experience of several different conditions of persons so the reader can assess how care might be provided by another and still maintain the level of love and compassion that they want for their loved one. Providing care is not a new phenomenon, with nuclear families that lived in the same area, older aging parents simply moved into the homes of their children and care continued. In the society of modernity, children have moved out of state and care has been subordinated to nursing and other adult care agencies. Care for older, aging family members has become a complex experience that requires spiritual understanding and physical training and abilities.

If you are seeking care for family you will want to read this book to better understand the demands and needs of care providers. After reading this book, persons in the health care field and in our faith based organizations may seek to pull together partnerships to provide care. Pastor Turner has positioned this care within a faith based context as a means of continuing the ministry of Jesus Christ. Jesus said in (Matthew 25:40 KJV) Inasmuch as ye have done it unto one of the least of these my brethren, ye have done it unto me. When a person becomes involved in the care of another human being, they have moved into the fulfillment of what Jesus desires that we love one another. This book is a method whereby you can become the vessel that God uses to make the environment your loved one experiences more loving and compassionate.

This caring subject matter invades my heart again and again with remembrances of my dear mother who journeyed these mundane shores via hospice and our loving hands. We have our respite now, nevertheless, sweet memories linger on Mother.

Reverend Floyd A. Davis
Twelfth Street Missionary Baptist Church

REVEREND DAVIS CREDENTIALS

THE REVEREND FLOYD A. DAVIS has been serving as pastor of the Twelfth Street Missionary Baptist Church since February 1, 2004. Prior to that he served as the pastor of the St. Francis Missionary Baptist Church for 10 years. His educational background includes an honorary Doctorate in Divinity from the Tennessee School of Religion, a Master in Theology from the Tennessee School of Religion, a Masters in Business Administration from Columbia University, a Bachelor in Technology from the University of Dayton, and 35 hours of Seminary Training toward the Master of Arts with a major in Biblical Studies at Ashland Theological Seminary.

Reverend Davis professional experiences, in addition to his pastoral duties include beginning in 1972 - Selected as an Administrative Intern for the Woodrow Wilson Foundation serving as Assistant to the Business Manager at Spelman College; Served as a Systems Analyst for the Burroughs Corporation; Served as a Programmer Analyst for the Advance Mortgage Corporation; Served as Programmer Analyst for the Ford Motor Company in various assignments; Served as Senior Programmer Analyst for the Occidental Petroleum Company; Served as Senior Consultant for the Systems International, Inc; Served as an Independent Contractor to many small businesses helping with the development, installation and maintenance of personal computer systems. As an independent consultant, in cooperation with Drew School of Los Angeles, he served the University of Kinshasa in Zaire, Africa with the selection, installation and operation of a personal computer to analyze demographic data.

In November 1984, Reverend Davis was found to be a "man of good report", "full of the Holy Ghost", and he was appointed over the work of the Kingdom to be a Deacon where he served until 1988. In 1986 he acknowledged the Call and Claim of Christ upon his life and began studying for the Gospel Ministry. In April 1986 he was ordained a Deacon and walked out of the ranks of the Board of Deacons and into the Gospel Ministry. In May 1988 he was licensed to preach the Gospel and in June 1990 he was ordained. Rev. Davis is a devoted family man. He has a wife, Odessa of 27 years, two sons, and one daughter.

ISAAC TURNER'S THOUGHTS

The kernel of insight was generated in one of Dr. B. Wayne Hopkins orientation meetings regarding the Master of Arts Research Field Project. I was mentally considering a ministry to "Boys with Behavioral Problems" or "Ministry to Blind, Deaf and Dumb Persons" or "Ministry to Developmentally Delayed Persons". The latter impressed me more as I thought how we would facilitate such ministries. I determined the other two were realistically future. As I thought on the human resources, the availability of skilled persons in my congregation dictated this was the best route and the Christian service rendered would be momentous. I knew I needed to be two years ahead in planning (and its good I did) to have the project off the drawing board and into service. I began reading all the literature I could on the subject of Respite Care. From local libraries and colleges and universities around the country and from Respite agencies, I read and received inspiration that the project was ripe and right for our Church. Although it is well documented that the Developmentally Delayed Persons are seemingly in an umbilical cord relationship with their parents, providers, or caretakers, yet it did not take much observation to discern that a rest was needed. The rest I speak of is needed by the caring persons. This is so because it is the parents or caretakers that are hurting in mind and spirit. They have been overwhelmed by the demands of the care recipient. There is this constant drain on the physical and mental energies because of the ever present responsibility to encourage, train, wash, feed, monitor, and evaluate their loved one.

For these and countless other reasons, I felt the Christian Church ought to be on the cutting edge of Respite Care Ministries. Are we not called of God to demonstrate and illustrate with our personhood and energies the many examples to alleviate suffering left heritage to us by the scripture record (2 Kings 4:26; 1 Pet. 5:7; Phil. 2:25-28; 1 Cor. 12:25, 26; Luke 10:34, 35; Acts 14:8-10). God has a will for the Developmentally delayed and physically delayed person and part of that will is that they be cared for and that the caring person has time for rest -- we must soften our hearts (Ex. 8:15, 31:15). The term "Respite" means "Rest". We give rest to the provider and both provider and the Care Recipient are benefited.

Therefore, this project is undertaken to perform and aide others in doing likewise to care for disabled persons with a quality Respite Care under Christian auspices.

CONTENTS

INTRODUCTION

How I wish this need for Respite Care could be emblazoned in the shopping centers across our nation because Respite Care is in the land, yet many are closing down either because people are not aware of its presence or parents do not trust their treasures with strange organizations. Respite Care among other things is any period of temporary relief or rest from parenting responsibilities. Families can and do receive relief because of its ministries. Some Respite Care facilities are funded, others like ours are gratuitous. Some are provided by friends, relatives, skilled care providers, or even professionals in the home of the Care Recipient or in another location. We utilize both the home, church and other locations. Our care is provided for one hour to three hours at present. When there is an emergency, we will extend the time limit.

Our Respite Care is occasional and also on a regular basis to any type family which has a chronic illness or disability. Our Respite Care Program has been found to be a part of the overall support system that families need to maintain their loved ones at home and the need of periodic rest for themselves. It is our observation that all parents and caretakers, whether of healthy persona or those with special needs, need quiet time away from daily responsibilities. So it seems care providers for disabled persons need this service and break even more. We observed the extra demands upon the caretaker by the Care Recipients. Special medical, physical, emotional, and educational needs make our Respite Care Program a needed part of such families' lifestyle. Sadly, many caretakers say they feel guilty about seeking help and using Respite Care. They are under the burden of feeling they should be able to manage all of their recipients' care. They don't want to be perceived as inadequate parents. What we try to instill in the caretaker is that time spent away from people with special needs is most important for the caretaker and the rest of the family. Each Care Recipient's needs are special; therefore, this impact on the family should be minimized. The family needs to take advantage of Respite facilities. We are here to help in the name of the Lord Jesus. At times the needs of the Care Recipients seem overwhelming; therefore, our Respite Care Services comes to the rescue.

We recommend to the churches of the nation to get involved in the Respite Care Ministry. Heavenly rewards accrue for those who bind up the wounds of His little lambs (Luke 10:34). We trust there is something in this written work project that will encourage and inspire persons to engage themselves in this most meaningful ministry. Your helping hand will minimize the cries of the lambs.

Caring for a child with special needs challenges both the Church, the families of the Care Recipient and the Care Giver. This can be the crowning achievement of your Christian commitment. Yes, the demands may seem overwhelming at times, but a break from these demands revitalizes your energy, broadens your perspective and restores your lost sense of humor. Check it out for yourself, this caring ministry restores your joy. Respite care is a fresh breath of oxygen to the caretakers who need all the assistance they can get. Don't forget about this "forgotten" segment of our society; the caretaking person who needs a respite.

The Scripture lifts up to us destitute persons and enjoins us to help hear those who stand in need (Prov. 31:8,9; 18:14; 17:22; 4:20-22; 3:7,8). Although Our Lord Jesus was not in the Respite ministry per se, yet He did let Mary rest (Luke 10:39-42) and He offered all those who were burdened and heavy laden a rest (John 21:10-12; Matthew 11:28). Jesus was about meeting crucial needs of humanity and we should be no less involved in lightening the heavy load humanity bears because of the curse of sin. The apostles John and Peter demonstrated their call to the caring ministry by stopping one day on their way to worship to make whole a suffering individual (Acts 3:1-8). It is the will of the Master that we be whole (Matthew 5:48). Our ministry helps the fractured toward wholeness -- sometimes at the expense of our suffering. But to suffer for one's own beliefs is integrity of the magnitude that produces health on both sides of the fence.

CHAPTER 1

THE FIELD PROJECT AND ITS BEGGING NEED

As we stood before God and this vast city void of respite care from churches, the vastness of the need impacted us. It goes without saying; the immensity of it all was overwhelming. The four of us met and prayed for guidance and success in a venture we felt the Lord would have us undertake. We discussed problems we might face and have to overcome including:

1. There was no record of another church having success in this area available to us.

2. The many services to the developmentally delayed persons rendered by the State of Georgia, County of Chatham and City of Savannah were void of specific church oriented respite care.

3. The social agencies were already over programmed and could not provide the kind of service we envisioned.

Other factors impacting us were:

1. Respite was an acknowledged need in our State.

2. It was ascertained that our respite care would be a vital supportive service in actually keeping the family unit intact.

3. Our involvement could keep the recipient from being institutionalized for that period of time.

4. The dire need to alleviate the hurts and despondency of the families and Caregivers who are consistently overlooked.

5. The potential exhilaration for having stood in the gap where heretofore no one volunteered to assume this position of care.

This need to help the caregiver was easily overlooked because the handicapped and critically ill persons need always obliterated the crying need of the care provider. Now we have the whole picture, no shadows. Clear photo prints, the need was begging to be alleviated.

CHAPTER 2

GETTING READY PHASE

Yes, we saw the picture. The need was plainly observed. The challenge was before us. What should we do? The same as so many before us, that is pray about it until all is lost, or roll back our sleeves and get involved in the process to minister. It did not take much brainstorming to ascertain that a concept and approach must be strategized to avoid failure in the respite venture. We considered our greatest resource, a resource which all churches have in common, the resource of volunteer workers.

The Christian Church can almost always count on this compassionate empathetic and caring human resource being utilized when called upon. These strategies were established to actualize a smooth development of community working services. To initiate a level of trust and confidence between the church and the governmental social agencies, we had to establish a staff committee for implementation of staff policies. We designated this phase of our program to be a pilot program in metamorphosis; becoming through procedural transformation our vision.

At a staff meeting it was determined that staff members who were presently active in the care giving field would lead out in the development of policies using their expertise as advisors and policy makers, and also to work with the parents and caregivers in compiling a list of needs and expectations. It was decided to go beyond the boundaries of our local church to find volunteers qualified to serve in this care ministry.

The staff steering committee would:

1. Do the ground work of the pilot program.

2. Develop necessary forms for the ministry.

3. Develop an orientation session for respite caregivers.

4. Develop screening forms to evaluate volunteer workers.

5. Check out the needs for insurance and possibility of liability.

CHAPTER 3

TRIAL AND ERROR PHASE DOCUMENTATION WITH OVERVIEW OF POTENTIAL AND REAL PROBLEMS

One area in the Respite Care Program where there is potential and real problems is in the contact with the families of the Care Recipient. As we surveyed the families it became apparent that surveying these potential resources posed a potential problem. Families were not always ready to disseminate intimate information. We sometimes had to re-formulate questionnaires to accommodate the mind set of caretaking families. From case to case, there was variance that dictated to us to redefine the parameters of appropriate services time with statements of the minimum and maximum service periods offered. We had to develop service applications that would fit situational procedures and ascertain what service provisions might surface and suggest potential solutions. This brainstorming was sometimes fun and sometimes like bumping our heads against the wall.

Out of it came a bevy of forms and ideas we can select from to help accommodate various respite care. We found through trial and error that mismatching families with workers put the Respite Care service in jeopardy. This error was also experience in the personnel when there were personality clashes that rendered a minimum of productivity until the situation was reevaluated and a suitable adjustment was agreed upon. We determined it would be advantageous to have families sign liability releases. In this matter we consulted legal counsel. We agreed to present selected information about the program to the Church and public. The chair established the practice of periodic evaluation of services and providers and the practice of modifying the program as deemed needed. In our staff meetings we are always open to any special needs surfacing in the program with our special attention leaning toward suggestion guidance and other related concerns of the Respite Care Ministry. Let your target dates be flexible. Fixed and firmed dates can become frustrating as the date nears without program meshing. Documentation of problems and a time rationalization of these problems, usually minimize a continuation of error and give stability to the staffs sense of management.

CHAPTER 4

ESTABLISHING THE RESPITE CARE MINISTRY WITH IMPLEMENTATION, EVALUATION AND RECOMMENDATIONS (OUR WAY OF CARING)

On the pages of this chapter, you will see the methodology used by our Respite Care Service. We are not professionals per se, but we are caring paraprofessionals who endeavor to serve persons at an optimum level of credibility. If you learn a more correct way of performance by our documenting our failures and successes, we will have done humanity a dual service. We enjoy our labor of love. We come to its challenges with our outstretched arms and hands saying, "Lord make me a blessing today."

We began our meetings at Church, but we have found the home of one of our staff persons is more suitable and convenient to all involved. We began meeting in January weekly. The meetings were in the evening during the week. Then we changed directors and our new director preferred 8:00 a.m. meetings on Tuesdays. We had targeted a May start time. Before May, we had to curtail meetings to twice monthly. When May arrived, we had done as much administrative planning as was needed to start the Respite Care Ministry; nevertheless, we concluded that it would not be advantageous to begin the ministry in June or July. We therefore targeted September as the month of implementation. In September, we began our weekly meetings at 8:00 a.m.

on Tuesday and began the Church of God Respite Care Ministry for Mentally and Physically Developmentally Delayed Persons. We prayed for God's blessing on the ministry and its personnel. The excitement was obvious. In November we added another supervisor and her job demands dictated another change in our meeting schedule. Friday evenings at 6:00 p.m. became our weekly or bi-weekly staff meeting time.

In this chapter, you will find a selection of some of the respite caregivers and workers' routines, the expectancy, and the care productivity. We are pleased that our heavenly Father allowed us this variety of vineyard labor on our way to heaven.

Documentation of Actual Care Giving For: Jimmy Holmes

Caretaker - Joseph Young

Caregiver - Joan Fuller

Care Recipient - Jimmy Holmes

Respite Schedule - Thursday 4:00 - 7:00 pm

Place - Home of Caretaker

Duties - Varied each week. To continue assistance in helping teach changes in abnormal behavior and to give other care and activity assistance as needed during the three hours of Respite Care.

After a normal interview with Mr. & Mrs. Joseph Young, the applications were filled out at their home and a specified date was set for the Respite Care ministry to begin. Thursdays from 4:00pm to 7:00pm was selected as an appropriate time for all parties concerned. Thursday, September 5, 1991 was targeted. Thursday at 3:45pm, I arrived at their home. I was received with smiles of anticipation by Mr. & Mrs. Joseph Young. We sat down in their living room and they instructed me of what they expected of me for the next three hours. They were very specific in what they wanted done for the Care Recipient Jimmy Holmes, an incapacitated sub teenager who was severely retarded physically and mentally unable to walk or talk. He moved by crawling or scooting around on his hands and knees. Jimmy and I hit it off as friends right away. After Mr.& Mrs. Joseph Young made their exit, I began by performing some of the motor skills helps they had itemized. I began by teaching Jimmy how to get on and off the bed by himself. He had a bed that helped this procedure. It was a handmade, fourteen and a half inch indentured bed with a mattress. A ramp was built on to facilitate Jimmy to crawl up and down to the bed by himself. My care was helped by the fact that because the bed was new to Jimmy, it was exciting for him to learn to use it. I worked with him to help him move to different positions on the bed. Each time he performed satisfactorily, I chimed, "Good boy." I taught and retaught him to turn on his right and left side. Each time he did so, he got a "good boy" affirmation from me. After a while, each "good boy" from me yielded a cooing smile from him. He was enjoying himself and the attention he was getting. I must confess, I was enjoying his positive responses to my teaching overtures. After the first hours, I moved on to helping him just simply lie on his back and stomach and to pull himself up in a sitting position. Then I was able to say to Jimmy, "Let's get off the bed," and show him how to lie down on the side of the ramp. I said, "Good boy, Jimmy, now let's turn over on your stomach, good, now let's get off the ramp." He got down off the ramp with my help. I was thinking, he was responding well with his motor skills. Now would be a good time to assist him in undressing. We have found teaching children to undress is easier than teaching them to dress. Of course, there is a lot of repetition in the teaching process which demands patience and kindness from the care giver. To help him learn and relearn the motor actions to remove his shirt, I had to use graduated guidance (hand over hand). This procedure was done thusly:

1. Place dormant hand on the back of his neck over the neck of the shirt, pull bottom of the shirt up to the neck.

2. Pull the shirt up to his head and then over his head.

3. Practice transferring his hands to pull the sleeves off.

In all these procedures, I made sure Jimmy assisted me as I assisted him. It was rewarding watching him put on his shirt. What was so easy for me was laborious for him, but he got so much satisfaction out of doing each little procedure. He slowly raised his foot to put on his briefs, then his knee pads, and alternately his pants, socks and shoes. Of course, some of these procedures he did well from practice, but it's like taking daily exercise. Some things have to be practiced over and over, even when they have already been done for the day. Jimmy had to position his feet and body in a special way to put on his briefs and pants. This was done in this manner: He placed his feet flat on the bed with his legs propped up to raise his body. He alternately raised his foot (right and left) to put on socks and shoes. There was almost always this need to point up the procedures. What he had learned previously was good, but this practice was supportive of the daily routine of being semi-independent with certain motor skills. With those teachings and reinforcement practices done, we went into the family room to play and watch T.V. until the caretakers returned. The Youngs were about fifteen minutes late but very joyful when they checked and noticed Jimmy's happy face. I informed them I had followed their written instructions and Jimmy has responded well. I affirmed the appointment for next Thursday and I was out of there with a smile and a feeling of a job well done for the Master caregiver.

Second Respite Care Ministry

Thursday evening, September 12, I arrived at 3:55pm. Once I entered the home, I could see the Youngs had readied Jimmy for dinner, but he had not been fed yet. The dinner was ready on the stove. I told the couple to leave and I could readily finish setting the table and serve Jimmy his dinner. They were going out to dinner and I told them to enjoy it. I took this opportunity to check out Jimmy's habits and abilities at the dinner table. I had him scoot himself up to the table and then I slid the hogg chair under him, so he was seated at the table thusly. I then gently placed his right hand on his lap. With this done, I rolled his chair under the table. Then I very carefully and patiently had him repeat "sounds of grace" before he began eating. It was now my challenge to get Jimmy to eat with a minimum of spills. Of course, he had to be bibbed. There was an adaptive (built up handle for his handicap) spoon and scoop for picking up some food. This was tedious, but he was able to accommodate himself. His plate was also an adaptive (indentured) plate, so the spoon could fit under the side and not fall off. I had to remind him of little simple things such as, "Put your spoon in your mouth, Jimmy. Now chew your food good." I found that encouraging him to chew worked well. On that day I was able to help him learn to use his adaptive cup and sit it on the table. It came to my mind how the Lord had said "When I was hungry, you fed me" (Matthew 25:35). He was not the only one that was beaming. I was not as successful in teaching him to grasp the handle of an adaptive metal handle with a screw to tighten the belt around his cup. I determined that in subsequent care visits, I would work on this chore when the opportunity presented itself. Jimmy demonstrated greater success at picking up the cup, drinking and setting it on the table. He had previously been assisted in this drink routine. He liked the table manners grace of using a table napkin. The napkin became many things to him (a flag, a fan, a bird, a nose blower and a dish towel). With all of these game distractions, you wonder how he learned to pick up the napkins (hand over hand) and carry it to his mouth and wipe it clean, but he did. I helped him practice the wiping of his mouth over and over again. When his meal was completely consumed and he intimated he was full or satisfied, I proceeded to assist him in leaving the table. Almost every effort was a learning or re-learning experience, and as long as he showed no fatigue, he seemed to enjoy the exercise. To make him feel useful, I asked him to push off from the table while I pulled the hogg chair back from the table while he was sitting in it. He grunted as if he was putting great effort into the exit from the table. This was quite an effort for Jimmy, it entailed:

1. Leaning over to the table

2. Standing up as best he could in his deformed condition

3. Kneeling to kneel down

4. Crawling away from the table

5. Putting the napkin in the trash can in the kitchen

Every little effort he made by himself was vital in his feeling useful and a contributor in the household. I proceeded to wash the few dinner dishes and let Jimmy hold the drying towel for me. With that exercise completed, we retired to the family room where we played patty cakes his style. When the caretakers returned, I informed them dinner went well, and that Jimmy even helped me with the dishes by holding the drying towel for me. They expressed their gratitude for me giving them a completely free hour to look in each others' eyes and simply talk. I confirmed the Respite Care ministry for next Thursday and I was off the case.

Third Respite Care Ministry

Thursday, September 19, I arrived at 3:45pm. The Youngs were ready to go. They informed me there were some items on sale at the Oglethorpe Mall and they wanted to shop and browse and just sit in the promenade and watch the shoppers stroll by while they rested their feet over an ice tea and lemonade. It sounded good to me. Mrs. Young informed me Jimmy had been lacking in his toilet training performance, and if I could refresh his memory and performance, she would appreciate it. She was elated over the improvement in his table manners. I said, "Thank you kindly - it's my joy to assist, and Jimmy is so easy to work with." After they left, I got down on the floor of the family room with Jimmy and talked and laughed with him. We were friends by now and I knew how important it was to reinforce this feeling of camaraderie. I knew that once this link was established, it was vital that I appear on my regular appointment, for the Care Recipient feels they have ownership in you. It becomes important to sustain this feeling of trust and almost a dependency on your respite care visit. We played childish fun games for about an hour, then I told Jimmy we were going to practice toilet training and asked if that would be o.k. He made a funny guttural noise that I took for a trusting acceptance of my change in activity. I walked and Jimmy scooted and crawled to the bathroom. Let me assist you in your thinking so you can scrutinize this procedure. With Jimmy it was a piece of cake, because he had most of his act together thusly:

1. Jimmy could go to the bathroom via crawling.

2. He could turn on the light.

3. He could stand at the sink (on his knees).

4. He could move to the commode and sit down (I have to place my arms under his arms and walk him to the toilet to be seated).

5. He could get off the toilet by leaning forward on the transfer chair in the bathtub. He could then pull himself up and kneel down and crawl away.

Jimmy had developed a problem of starting too late for the bathroom and there was not enough time to negotiate his unclothing before his elimination started. We practiced hurrying from different locations in the house to the toilet. After a few times of helping him motivate in an expeditious manner, he seemed to sense the urgency of hurrying. Then he would hurry as if it was a "Special Olympics" race. I would say, "Time," and he would be off. When he disrobed his pants and briefs in an expeditious manner, I would show excitement and say, "Good boy, Jimmy, good boy, you made it," and give him a big hug. When he slowed, I would shake my head and say, "Try, try again." After a while, I sensed a minimal of success. Mrs. Young later informed me he started blurting out something before his toilet trek and scooted off to the toilet, and that his timing was improving. I told her he was trying to mimic me by saying "time" in an un-worded way. The ministry was again a delight that day. We set the next Thursday as our appointed time. I assessed the three hours as well spent and utilized in helping Jimmy in his motor skills and elimination processes. It was evident we were succeeding in not only giving the Youngs a needed rest, but also helping them use the time wisely to strengthen their marriage relationship by making it a quality time, as well as respite time.

Fourth Respite Care Ministry

Thursday, September 27, I arrived at 3:45pm. The Youngs were smiling and ready to go visit relatives. They asked me to assist Jimmy in eating his dinner which was already served and he was at the table eating. They gave me no other instructions. I sat and watched Jimmy and affirmed him, as he very carefully followed all the helpful instructions I had given him and helped him with previously. He even added an utterance which I took to be an expression of gratitude when I poured him another half glass of milk. I was a happy observer of a young boy who was developmentally and physically delayed but showing a substantial amount of progress in his memory retainment and physical motor skills. After dinner, I washed dishes and he held the drying towel. I gave him a couple of plastic saucers to dry, and he did. We retired to the family room for patty cakes and the old stand by T.V. When the Youngs returned, we were both showing signs of heavy eyelids and a kinship to Morpheus. The Youngs returned saddened by some of the deaths and sicknesses in the family, yet rejoicing because they got to sit and chat with loved ones who were somewhat neglected because of lack of time to visit. I chimed out as I made the next appointment for next month.

Fifth Respite Care Ministry

October 3, I arrived at 3:50pm and found the Youngs a bit pensive. They were going to a political rally for the female republican who was running against an entrenched mayor (20 year incumbent) on a platform to minimize the city's dope traffic and to drastically cut down on the murder rate in our city and bring again excellence in government administration. I bid them farewell after they gave me note of what I might try to accomplish in the three hours of respite care. They were really up to date on the teaching and learning aptitudes of persons with limited activities. I was glad I had been trained in this area and had years of background involvement in this field of compassion for those less fortunate. I was so thrilled when my church started the plans for the Respite Ministry the first part of the year. That night my assignment was to help Jimmy in his abilities to communicate. I began the activity by attempting to help him learn to listen better. I put my four fingers on Jimmy's ear and said, "Jimmy can listen with his ears." I then placed Jimmy's four fingers on his ear and said again, "Jimmy can listen with his ears." Then I spoke softly into one ear. I was attempting to help him practice listening with his ears. I began speaking softly close to him. Then I spoke softly from a short distance. Finally I repeated the whole process several times until I felt he was responding positively.

Next, I worked on his eye contact. I began with a soft light thusly:

1. I focused it between his eyes.

2. Then I looked closely and to see if I saw my eyes in his eyes.

3. I checked for eye movement. I moved an object from right to left and then
up and down. I repeated all of the above a few times. Jimmy responded well.

His last exercise was to check his response to his name thusly:

1. "Jimmy, Jimmy," I called.

2. I looked for an eye contact in response.

3. I then moved Jimmy's head and leaned his ear towards me and placed my four
fingers on his ear and vocalized, "Jimmy, Jimmy, my sweet Jimmy. Jimmy can
hear, Jimmy can listen." His response was positive. We repeated this exercise one
more time with better response.

I had time to evaluate the evening's encounter before the Youngs returned. I
was elated as I thought of all the handicapped persons with whom I had not had as
much success. I believe the Lord was encouraging me to stay in this ministry the rest of
my life. For such a severely handicapped boy, Jimmy was remarkably intelligent for his
age and development. All he needed was more of the kind of love and affection he was
getting from his caretakers.

When I thought about the power of love to restore sanity and physical
disabilities of twisted limbs and undeveloped voice and tongue apparatus, I just broke
down in tears of joy. Poor Jimmy didn't know what was happening and I just hugged
him and rocked him to let him know everything was all right, and that the love was still
flowing.

When the Youngs returned that evening, I didn't tell them they had set the stage
for me to worship the Lord in my spirit. They were now showing enthusiasm for the

female candidate for mayor of Savannah, Georgia. As they expressed themselves, I pulled on my sweater and made the appointment for next week, still under the afterglow of the sweet visitation of the Lord Holy Spirit.

The Sixth Respite Care Ministry

October 10, I arrived at the Youngs at 3:45pm. They were still undecided as what to do with their respite. Mrs. Young wanted to go to the recreation park and take in the fall colors as the trees and bushes changed from green to the vivid colors of fall. Mr. Young wanted to go to a tent revival meeting at 5:30pm. They asked me to help them in their thinking. I told them that since the idea of the respite was to have a peaceful three hours, I thought some hamburgers, french fries, shakes and a walk through the nature trail amid all God's creative beauty would be a fitting setting for an evening worship just for the two of them. Mr. Young hesitantly agreed. They dressed warmly although it was 72 degrees outside. They left no directives, this time and I didn't come with a planned evening. I greeted Jimmy who hugged me as best as he could. This gave me an idea. I said, "Jimmy, let's socialize this evening, come on. Let's begin by touching objects. See here, touch like I do." I began touching unbreakable objects. "See," I began touching the chairs and tables. I took his hands and did the same with them and then he had it. A funny smile came on his face and he began to scoot behind me touching everything I touched. Then I changed to feeling the objects, and Jimmy began feeling the objects with that funny sound he makes when he is content and happy. After that we changed to a "seeing" game and from that to a "hearing" game. We even tried a "smelling" game. We soon went through the five senses and we had fun. We tried sitting alone, and we tried running for me and crawling fast for Jimmy. Then we went out in the yard and tried rolling and hitting the plastic ball. Suddenly I wondered where this energy came from. With that thought, I resorted to my crutch. I said, "Let's go in the house and play a game on TN." We went in to the one eyed distraction, and I explained we were going to play "laugh." We just made almost everything funny and laughed and he made some new happy sounds while we played. We added to that "happy" body movement. We ended it all with a hug and a kiss. The boy had a strong embrace for a physically handicapped fellow. I literally had to peel his arms out from around me. When the Youngs returned, they could tell we had a good time because we were beaming. The Youngs looked like two people in love. I don't know whether the outdoor devotion or the colors of the leaves or maybe both had prompted the "love" look. We said good night, with a respite date for next Thursday. I really looked forward to the Thursday respite care ministry.

As I look at this respite care ministry in regard to Mr. & Mrs. Joseph Young and Jimmy Holmes, I see progress in that we helped the Youngs get their needed rest, and we achieved the assigned goals. We helped Jimmy change some abnormal behaviors through positive reinforcement of each activity such as:

1. To help him gain some independence in motor skills

2. To help Jimmy develop some self-help skills

3. To help him with toilet training

4. To reinforce positive table manners

5. To reinforce good eating habits

6. To help Jimmy learn to communicate better

7. To help him improve his social skills

8. To reinforce all activities with positive responses and gestures

The bottom line is that we helped Jimmy achieve these motor skills and self-worth and a maximum of confidence, and respite for the caregivers.

Respite Care Ministry of: Sherri Peters

Caretaker: Abraham Peters

Care Giver: Lois F. Bangs

Care Recipient: Sherri Peters

Respite Schedule: Periodically

Place: Home of care recipient and others

Duties: To counsel Sherri by phone and in person. To take and assist her in shopping. To pick her up when we have a Respite Care meeting and affair at the church.

History: Sherri was incapacitated at birth. I had the privilege of meeting Sherri twenty-two years ago when I was a trainer for the Chatham Association for Incapacitated Children. She was there being trained to work in a job setting program. Sherri was a very beautiful and sensitive young woman with a warm and winsome smile. She also was very trusting of everyone that she was around, and that sometimes led to problems for her especially so with men. Time after time male friends took advantage of her good and trusting nature. She was so easy going, and it was natural for her to trust and believe anything a so-called friend told her. Sherri was looking for true love, but all the system seem to dish out to her was sexual love and this of a low caliber. Sadly, Sherri didn't know the difference. She was often in tears and very confused about relationships. Her work performance was often hampered by the rending of her heart. She was walking around in a total state of confusion. Some young man would offer her friendship and propose an answer to her troubles. Sadly, part of the answer was always becoming a bed partner with the "doctor." We did what we could for the young confused lady, but there was very little we could do. It is hard to reason with a normal person in love. Retarded love must be multiple times harder to treat with maximum of success. I lost contact with Sherri for about fifteen years until, low and behold, she surfaced one Sunday and joined the Church where I was a member. I remembered Sherri as a very hard worker who always followed instructions well and was promoted to assistant to the cooks at the school cafeteria.

Sherri is an African-American of thirty-nine years old. She is married to Abraham Peters, who is also her caretaker. Sadly, her choices historically have continued to be destructive. Her husband is abusive. She has a history of being sexually and mentally abused by family and friends. Someone might label her as a loser since childhood. Her husband is considerably older than she and role models as a father-image. She repeatedly states that he is mean to her.

My Respite Care Ministry with Sherri began on November 6, 1991 with a telephone conversation with an overture for the ministry. Sherri was positive for help and her husband was open for the rest provided by our ministry. Sherri had just been released from Georgia Regional Rehabilitation Hospital (a state of Georgia Mental Institution) and as such, she was heavily medicated to keep her tranquilized. Before I could arrange a Respite Date, she was again hospitalized on November 13, 1991. I made contact with her there and again after she was released from Georgia Regional. She was much better this time. She was more in control of her voice even though she again was heavily medicated. On November 28, 1991, she was better and able to help me plan an outing for the both of us in early December. We planned to take care of any errands she needed to take care of and to have lunch together. She called me back to wish me a Happy Thanksgiving Day. On December 10, 1991, Sherri and I met her mother and some other relatives at the grocery store. We all had a brief fellowship and agreed to make contact for a monthly meeting and outing. Repeatedly, our December outing was canceled due to illness. Then my work schedule changed. During December and January, we often talked on the phone. She had been having dental problems. I coaxed her into seeing a dentist for her teeth care. She agreed to make a dental appointment for January 25 when I could provide transportation for her. We made definite plans for an outing after her dental work was completed. We planned to go to the breakfast at the Church for the Respite Care Program Workers and Care Recipients. We are all looking forward to this event in two weeks. Pastor Turner is cooking, the Care Providers are serving, and we are all eating and fellowshipping.

Respite Care Ministry Of: Mary Miller

Caretaker: Reverend Gus Miller

Caregivers: Beulah Baul and Ludene Kent

Care Recipient: Mary Miller

Respite Schedule: Varied and occasional and upon request.

Place: Home of Care Recipient

History: Mary Miller is a victim of senility which effects her motor reflexes and mind. She is blind and unable to care for herself. Her husband is partially incapacitated and in need of help himself, but because of pride, he refuses assistance.

Respite Care Ministry: Every Wednesday in November, Ludene Kent cooked and prepared hot meals for Reverend and Mrs. Miller. She also washed and dried their clothes. On other days as solicited or requested, she took dinners as a part of Respite Care and stayed with Sister Miller while Reverend Miller ran errands and shopped.

Every Wednesday in December, the Respite Care Ministry fed the Millers and Sister Ludene Kent sat with Sister Mary Miller, singing and praying, while Reverend Miller was freed up to run needed errands for his household.

In January, Beulah Baul and Ludene Kent rendered Respite Care to Mary Miller with additional service, cleaned house and did other needed chores. Reverend Gus Miller who has recovered from a prostate cancer operation, was freed up to leave and go shopping, and other needed business was taken care of during the Respite Care two hours. Also during the month, whenever the need presented itself, Sister Ludene Kent took care of her financial transactions (bills, banks, utility payments, etc.).

Continuation of Respite Care Ministry of: Leola Sanders

Caretaker: Leola Sanders

Caregivers: James Baul

Care Recipient: Leola Sanders

Respite Schedule: November, December, January. Varied times, when needed.

Place: Home of Recipients and Others

History: Mrs. Sanders is an elderly widow who asked for help from our Respite Care Ministry when she had no transportation to and from the hospital. This resulted in a continuing ministry after she was dismissed from the hospital. This case varies from our usual acceptance roster; nevertheless, since we had an available caregiver who wished to assist, we became involved.

In November, Mrs. Leola Sanders requested transportation to the hospital from our Respite Caregiver, James Baul. He did so and when she was released, she asked for transportation again and was given transportation home.

In December, while recuperating, the ministry continued in the form of paying her bills, doing her shopping, and mailing her parcels.

In January, the care continued and increased to transport her to her physician for her medical check-ups. The care ministry will continue until the patient is well enough to handle her own affairs.

Respite Ministry to: Ulysses Grant

Respite Caretakers: Mr. & Mrs. K. David (Sadie) Dawkins

Respite Caregiver: Reverend Isaac C. Turner

Recipient: Ulysses Grant

Respite Schedule: September 21, 1991 - 10:00 a.m.- 1:00 p.m.

After Greeting Mr. King David Dawkins, and inquiring about recipient, I found the recipient was not fully groomed. His unreadiness was no barrier. The caretaker helped complete his grooming and brought him out. I asked if he had a sweater or jacket as the morning weather was unusually cool and windy (68 degrees). A jacket was secured. After greeting Ulysses, we drove off to Burger King to get six "Buddy" breakfasts, two large coffees, and some jelly. We drove fifteen miles to Tybee Island to the beach where we got out and found a log where we could sit and eat our breakfast. While the waves crashed in and the sea gulls played and flew around us, we ate and talked. He was most cheerful and hungry. After I had listened and let him talk for an hour, we walked a mile down the beach and picked up small sea shells. I chimed about the wonders of God creating oceans for fish to swim in and surfers to glide on. Of course, he out walked me. After he collected his shells, I gave him mine. He was all smiles. I finally had to say, "Let's head back to the car." He could not stop saying what a good time he was having. We drove back to the city with the same happy chatter. His mom and step-dad were waiting and grateful for the break. We exchanged pleasantries and said our farewells for this respite encounter, which by God's grace had been well done. P.S. There is more to tell.

On the way home from the beach, the "retarded" brother was putting the con on me and I was not aware of his mental alertness. He spoke with a stutter and lisp, nevertheless, he was leading me on to a point he had already set his mind on. First, he admired my watch. Then he said he liked watches and that he had one, but recently it broke and did not keep time any more. Ulysses asked me if I had another watch. I said I did. He then asked me what I did with it. I told him it was at home in a drawer, because the wrist band was broken. He asked me if I was going to have it fixed. I told him it was the kind that was welded into the watch and could not be replaced. He then asked me if it kept good time. Again I said it did. He then had me where he wanted me and said, "You outta give me the watch". "Don't you think I need a watch?" He had me! I said, "Yes, you can have the watch." He reacted like a child at Christmas and asked me when. I said, I would bring the watch to Church the following Sunday. Sunday, his mother had him cleaned up and in Church. Right after Sunday School he hobbled over to me and asked, "You, you got my watch?" I took the watch out of my pocket and gave it to him. He reacted as a child who had received a bike; all smiles, all giggles. It was a good way to end a Respite care encounter.

Respite Ministry to: Mrs. Sadie Dawkins

Respite Caretakers: Mrs. Sadie Dawkins

Respite Caregiver: Reverend Isaac C. Turner

Recipient: Ulysses White

Respite Schedule: October 3, 1991

Place: Home of the respite care recipient

After our jail ministry at the Chatham County Jail 9 a.m. to 11 am, I went to keep the appointment I had previously made with Mrs. Sadie Dawkins, the parent of Ulysses White. I had secured her approval to rest her that day from the routine of caring for her son Ulysses. She was elated when I called her and reminisced of the last respite care rendered to her family. She now had three men at home, all disabled. Ulysses was born with retardation and other physical ailments such as deformity in both legs, yet he was able to walk on twisted feet. His hands were also twisted. His speech was hard to understand because of speech defects. The other two men were more pitiable: Billy and Seymour had both contracted the disease Aids. The disease was in various stages. Their Caretaker had opened her doors for them to come and be cared for by her and her husband. I ministered to Billy the time I waited for Ulysses to come out of his room. Mrs. Dawkins is a "pack-rat" so there is clutter from the backyard through the whole house except in the bedroom. She sells second hand furniture for a living. Ulysses finally appeared with his happy toothy grin and asked me what I had for him today. I told him, "Just me and Jesus," but that we were going to the movie to see "The Adams Family," which was about a kookie family who had lost Mr. Addam's

44

brother for several years and they wanted to find him again. This pleased Ulysses and he said, "Good, I like that."

I asked him if he liked popcorn and he readily affirmed that. I told him we would have popcorn and soda. Mrs. Dawkins offered me $2.50 for treats. I refused, but she insisted, so I took the donation. We said goodbye and were off to the theater. I was strategizing in my mind how to keep up with Ulysses at the movies. He had gotten away from his mother in public places before and sometimes been gone for days. I purposely selected a theater that had unfamiliar surroundings. I had previously arranged with the manager for free passes and free popcorn. So now I had to figure out what to do with the $2.50. We went in and I had Ulysses sit down in the lobby while I approached the assistant manager for the refreshments. He waited on us himself with a barrel of popcorn and a large drink for each of us. With this secured, I asked Ulysses if he needed to go to the restroom (realizing this could be a possible escape point for him), but he said he didn't. We went into the theater and I purposely selected the back row, because I knew he talked in a higher pitched voice than normal people, that he might blurt out at any time, and that he possibly had to use the restroom facility. We sat and waited for the movie to begin. Ulysses chatted and told me about his "girlfriend" at the center for dysfunctional persons he attended daily. Daisy Sue was her name, and he and Daisy Sue made projects together and she teased him sometimes. You could tell these were happy times for him. He had commendable things to say about his supervisor. The movie was about to begin and I told him to be quiet. He became surprisingly quiet during the whole movie. He was steadily eating his popcorn, drinking his soda, and giving rapt attention to the film. When the film was little past half way, he suddenly stood up and said, "I have to go to the restroom." We hurriedly went to the men's room. Again I was on alert because I had to use one enclosed stall and he another, and I was fearful he might finish before me and start walking out. But he waited for me, and we washed and went out to spend the $2.50 on candy bars. We returned to the movie and again he sat quietly and attentively. I noted to myself, "We must do this again since the season is now cooling and not inclement for outdoor activity." When the movie was over, we started for the car and he showed no signs of trying to out-walk me or to escape. I asked him if he enjoyed the movie, and he said he had. I asked what part of the movie he liked best. Since it was a comedy, I thought he would select a funny sequence, but he said he liked the parts about the slides through the house down to the third basement and the one that led to the family graveyard best. On the way home, he thanked me for the watch and asked what else I had for him. I told him, "Sorry, but that was a one time gift. I don't have any other things to give away." He said, "Okay." When we arrived at his house, his parents had gone to their "re-sale" furniture shop. His brother Seymour was there and I talked to him about the good time we had in the outing. I told him that according to his mother's dictates, I would come again next month and give her a rest. She usually used Ulysses at the shop on Saturday to help around as best he could and would only need the Respite Care Ministry once a month and "on call" the rest of the time. I told my newly found "friend" I would take him out again in a few weeks and until then I would be seeing him periodically when his mother brought him to church. I told Seymour to take good care of Ulysses (both of the Aids patients were mobile and able to take long walks) and I was off to my schedule.

As I re-evaluated the Respite Care of Ulysses and the Respite Ministry to Mr. & Mrs. King David (Sadie) Dawkins, I am pleased with what has been accomplished and the ongoing ministry as well as with the addition of the Respite Ministry to our already successful ministry to Seniors. I feel we are showing a sense of maturation in Savannah in which we can be joyfully engaged in humane ministries beyond the four walls of the sanctuary. Out on the hedges, highway and by-ways of our community where the sheep are crying and bleating. I see nothing but positivity coming from the Respite Care Ministry. I can't wait until the Lord shows us another viable ministry with willing workers to facilitate the kingdom labor.

CHAPTER 5

OUR PROCEDURES

Our main concern here has been to maintain a level of care for the Care Recipient which is at the same level or higher than they are receiving at home. We have set policies reflecting that attitude. We feel obligated to be consistent with a high caliber of caring for persons entrusted into our care. Therefore, in our initial interview with the caretaker or care provider/parent we endeavor to establish these guidelines:

1. To let the caretaker alert us to standards and procedures expected of us from the caretaker.

2. To ask the caretaker for specifics of expectation from care recipients.

3. To simplify our policy to both the caretaker and the care recipient.

4. To check for eligibility of the recipient.

5. To establish the fact that any caretaker, parent, etc, who is responsible for the well being of a care recipient is eligible for our program if volunteers match work load.

6. Persons visiting our fair city are all eligible to request respite care for their care recipient.

7. Our first priority is our church membership.

8. The simple procedure is to contact a respite care director or a supervisor and interview him and ask him to fill out the needed forms appearing in this chapter.

Only certain forms need to be sent out as each case dictates its needs. Phone numbers will be provided to obtain additional information about our respite care program.

9. All respite care requests must be made using one of our designated numbers. All requests are documented for future reference.

10. All policies stated on forms or verbally must be compiled with for eligibility.

11. All forms are confidential and will be kept in closed files.

12. All files tendered to the potential consumer must be filled out either by the consumer or the interviewer.

13. The exception is emergency cases. In the event of emergency, forms may be filled out later.

14. The respite care agreement must be signed by the party responsible for the care recipient.

15. Failure to comply with our rules and procedures renders the consumer/ caretaker and care recipient ineligible for our care placement at that time.

16. Although transportation may be provided by our program, this is not guaranteed. The person requesting respite care shall be responsible for the care recipient's transportation.

17. We promote safe and adequate care which we hope will meet the social, physical and emotional needs of our consumers.

18. All parents/caretakers must cooperate with our respite care program.

19.   It shall be a reason for refusal of services if there is any prior conviction of

admission to or plain evidence of care recipient abuse, care recipient

battering, molestation or neglect by the applicant.

The supplementary forms found in Appendix 3 are presented here to round out

procedure and standard forms for present and envisioned future needs.

CHAPTER 6

OUR VOLUNTEER PERSONNEL RESPONSIBILITIES

God has all kinds of people who will stand in the "gap" if we define what the "gap" is and what the need in the gap is. There is a need for fractured persons to be accepted as whole persons. It is a special kind of humans who want to get involved so much in bringing isolated and developmentally delayed persons back into meaningful community. These persons long to be bridges over the isolation that the handicapped often experience. Perhaps they cannot do the complete job - but they can get involved and get the ball rolling. Usually these "gap" persons want to volunteer to help. We must find ways to capture their attention to the Respite Care Ministry and let them know we need them in this support group of ministering to persons much less fortunate than they. Our volunteer personnel responsibilities are set by the personal and systemic needs that develop within and without our Respite Care Program. We ask for loyalty to the Lord Jesus Christ and to His Kingdom programs. Did he not promise us rest for our souls while we labor for him in the flesh? (Matthew 11:29, 30). Was not our Lord committed to healing the mentally incapacitated and releasing them to witness of the goodness of the Lord Christ? (Luke 8:38, 39; Mark 5:18-20). Also, be loyal to the Respite Care Ministry and to the brothers and sisters who tend to this holistic ministry of caring and doing. Need I say more?

Although it is well documented that the Developmentally Delayed Persons are seemingly in an umbilical chord relationship with their parents, providers, or caretakers, it does not take much observation to discern that a rest is needed. The rest I speak of is needed by the caring persons. This rest is needed for various reasons, some of them are:

1. They are hurt in mind and spirit.

2. They have been overwhelmed by the demands of the care recipient.

3. The ever present responsibility to encourage, train, wash, feed,

    monitor and evaluate.

4. The constant drain on the physical and mental energies, etc.

These responsibilities and more can and do pose an overwhelming burden of near hopelessness when there is no planned and real rest. At this time, the nation and the church are becoming aware of this acute need. Therefore a Respite Ministry is in order for churches such as ours. The question is what form this noble idea will take and how we shall be about our Father's business so that His will for developmentally delayed persons will be administered.

This Respite Ministry Project is especially designed to aide care providers and developmentally disabled persons with a respite and care that will maintain dignity and love as we minister in this relief from daily responsibilities.

This need to help the caregiver was easily overlooked because the handicapped persons need always obliterated the crying need of the care provider. Now we had the whole picture--no shadows. Clear photo prints--the need was begging to be alleviated.

CHAPTER 7

WHAT WE ARE ABOUT AND WHY

Our philosophy here at the Church of God for laboring in the ministry to developmentally delayed persons is simply to express and act upon our concern for our families who have developmentally disabled persons living at home and need a rest. Our observation has been that these families are often tired and in need of help. Our program allows them occasional or periodic time off from the rigors and demands of caring for their handicapped person. Therefore, we have created a much healthier and wholesome atmosphere for the whole household. Our intervention holds back or eradicates "burn-outs" and gives hope to a parent or caretaker who otherwise might feel the cares of the whole retarded world resting on their shoulders. Already, we are receiving appreciative remarks both from parents and members of the congregation and we have just touched the water. Again and again, we observed several programs and this is understandable since their need is so glaring. Yet the rest of the family, who are also incapacitated, have limited ways of alleviating their needs. Therefore, we emphasize we are prioritizing the family although we are working with the handicapped person. This manifestation of caring for the caretaker has already shown a tremendous psychological power to heal. It frees (up) the family to admit they are hurting and in need of respite care. Healing on any level is beneficial to the handicapped member also.

We are continuing our caring ministry even though there are only five of us working now. We envision a greater volunteer participation, thereby allowing us greater access to the mounting need in our community. Although stressed out families in our local church helped us to see the respite care need, the need reaches far beyond the borders of our local church. If we can but be a toe in the pool of Siloam to prove the angel is indeed troubling the waters of respite care, so be it!

Procedures in Establishing a Respite Care Program

A major concern of families is the general lack of availability of respite care services. In many areas, there are no formal respite programs. For this reason, suggestions about how to start a respite program are included below:

- Survey the needs of the community

- Consider whether any existing programs or services can be restructured to meet families' needs for respite (for example, respite beds in hospitals, nursing homes, or group homes)

- Contact other respite programs and review written resource material

- Determine which type(s) of respite might be most suitable in the particular community

- Create network with parent groups and community groups serving

  In-home respite care

  Out-of-home respite care

  Residential facilities

      nursing homes

      pediatric hospitals

state institutions

Respite day care center

church facility

rehabilitation center

other day care setting

Group Homes

Foster Homes

Respite provider's home

Miscellaneous respite care

Recreation programs

Special camps

After-school programs

Comprehensive programs

In and out of home components

This networking began as a continuum of our in-home respite care, but soon broadened as an opening flower of respite care services. It seemed that the community and our church were ripe for our helping hand involvement. In fact, it made us wonder "What took us so long to center in on this need?" Jesus, our Lord, had sent everyone of us out into our community to care for needful humanity. Adding Respite Ministry to Soul Winning helps make a beautiful bouquet. Our Church Respite Team began with the immediate environ of our church families, nevertheless, we found our care was needed beyond our church confines. Some of our members were involved in city, county, and state facilities that had great outreach into pools of persons who were developmentally and physically incapacitated. We made contact with local facilities and the Chatham County Tideland Facility for Developmentally Delayed Persons.

As we considered the vastness of these patients, we zeroed in on an area that we could be of assistance. Of course careful scrutiny was given potential drivers and care relief givers. We then proceeded with our overture to the Tideland facility. Of course our ministry there varies from the home care. Nevertheless, the back bone is the same, caring for those in need of care, only there we pick up the care receivers and deliver them to a predestined place of recreation or workshop activity. In doing this, we are following an example set by Jesus Himself when He called seven of His disciples away from their labor of fishing and invited them to rest at a breakfast He had prepared for them (John 21:9-12). Thusly, because the need presented itself to us, we proceeded to begin a labor of love that manifested another of Respite Ministry to the glory of God.

Periodically, our Church gives this type of respite to the day caregivers at the Tideland facility. This respite is done on Sundays and it entails the preparing the Developmentally Delayed person to come to worship on Sunday morning. This worship is with the regular congregation. The congregation is prepared to assist the charges to enjoy the worship experience. The recipients are made to feel they are moving toward normalcy, when they participate in the worship experience, singing, praying, and sometimes giving vocal testimony to God's activity in their lives. This is the new procedure used throughout the nation (not to separate, but to include the care recipients in the community of the normal caregivers). This acceptance is working wonders. Many have been trained to work in supermarkets as baggers, janitors, etc. The pride and joy they bring to their employment is exciting to behold. They are courteous and effective in their job assignment. We try to enhance these attributes in our respite program. As much as is humanly possible, we let the recipients lead as they participate in the Saturday round of activities and as they testify to God's goodness in their lives during Sunday worship.

At a conference of staff members, Director Iona Brady suggested we broaden our focus to the physically Developmentally Delayed persons. Since we were somewhat already engaged in this pursuit, it seemed logical and ethical. We have several senior citizens who fit into this category being physically unable to attend church and care for themselves totally. Their caregivers surely needed a respite in their homes from the tedious load of caring and always needed to be near-by. We agreed to include the senior citizens who were incapacitated because of ill health, physically or mentally. Immediately we targeted three needful care recipient households. These were:

1. The Candler General Hospital Rehabilitation Unit. This research observed this unit's responsibility was to make patients comfortable while they were in confinement at the hospital. The staff goal was to take these discouraged persons and help them regain their courage and joy in living, to help them become and exhibit a newly found independence with special regards to their limitation, to get them prepared for their home going with a reasonable amount of dignity, to befriend patient by conversation and convincing them they are a viable part of society, and to contact outside relatives and friends. When the

57

patient is in severe pain and distress and medication does not remedy, verbal encouragement is administered where it is adaptable. Procedure in the morning is to make sure the patient is alert and adapting to his cause of rehab, which might be a stroke or other crippling diseases of mind or body. The goal is to re-teach them hygienic measure and how to dress and be as self-sufficient as possible, to help make the patient mobile using transfer techniques to wheel chair, to teach them to motivate safely in wheel chairs, to teach them how to walk again to gage them toward normalcy, to facilitate the catherization process, etc.

2. Interview at the home of David and Sadie Dawkins. Their son, Ulysses White, 49 years old, is a developmentally delayed person both physically and mentally. Ulysses, as we fondly call him, is handicapped in arm, hands, and legs and has a pronounced speech impediment. His demeanor is happy and he is outgoing although we are not always able to understand his speech. Ulysses runs away periodically in cold and hot weather and is later found in vicarious situations. Sometimes he returns home on his own. He likes to walk up and down the railroad tracks, which of course, causes his family great anxiety. He likes being outside, to ride and eat junk food. His mother is his main caregiver. We envision sharing some quality time with Ulysses.

3. Telephone contact was made with Ms. Carol Pope, the Assistant Principal of the Chatham-Effingham Psycho-Educational Facility on Cloverdale Streets. The principal is Mrs. Patsy Hinely. I was given an appointment to tour the facility.

This particular center specializes in educating the autistic children of our city. Many of these autistic children are severely handicapped by their retardation. This severity sets the stage for challenge and endeavor from the specialized staff of the Board of Education. Because of the severity of the retardation, it was decided that our staff would not have the expertise to effectively care for this type of patient.

We held a conference with the administrator Faythe Merkert, Chatham Association Center, 7211 Seawright Drive, P.O. Box 13662, Savannah, Georgia 31416. She led me on an enlightening tour of the vast resources of the center. It was very encouraging to see the positive involvements that caregivers can enter into with the recipients to better enhance their lifestyle daily, nurturing them and teaching them to become and maintain an adequate contributive lifestyle. It was determined that this was the level of mental and physical retardation that we could handle restoratively and beneficially both to the recipient and the caregiver.

At another staff meeting planned for the families and caregivers to document and consider their input, these helpful adjunctive services were mentioned as needful and helpful:

1. Parent support groups

2. Parent workshops on aspects of the care recipients care

3. Social events to bring families together

4. Discussion groups with parents and respite providers to encourage joint problem solving

5. Baby-sitting for siblings

6. Caregivers to accompany families on outings to help care for the recipient

7. Brief relief for parents when recipient is hospitalized

8. Before and after school care and summer daycare

9. A centralized respite referral agency or clearing house

Yes, we are about our Father's business of caring and acting out heaven's melodrama here on earth. Won't you please join us on your way to heaven? Here is one key to the Kingdom of Respite Care.

TERM DESIGNATIONS

Chair: The person who acts as chairperson of the staff and planning meetings.

Developmental Delayed: Refers to disabilities attributable to mental retardation, cerebral palsy, epilepsy, autism or any other neurological handicapping condition closely related to mental retardation and requiring treatment similar to that required by mentally retarded persons, if the disability originates before the individual reaches age 18, has continued or can be expected to continue indefinitely and constitutes a substantial handicap of the person. Or physical or mental impairment caused by old age (geriatrics).

Director: The person or persons in charge of the church related respite care program.

Family Support Service: Refers to services which enable the client's family to maintain the client in his natural homesitting. This service is intended to support the family, not supplant it.

Parents/Caretakers: Refers to parents or responsible persons providing care from a 24 hour day, seven days a week involvement with an individual who is developmentally disabled.

Placement: Refers to the time during which the developmentally disabled person is given respite care while the parent is away. Each respite care placement may range from one hour to 3 hours unless the need for extended care can be documented and approved by the Respite Care Staff.

Respite Care: Refers to a service provided to a developmentally disabled person whose primary need is a short-term care arrangement (in-home or out-of home) for planned or emergency needs. It may be provided for reasons of crisis assistance to the individual and family, family outing, and/or interim living arrangements, both to give the caretaker a needed rest and to accommodate the care recipient for a period of time. This care is directed toward maintenance of the developmentally disabled person in his family home or at church or on an outing (mall, picnic, etc.), although in some cases respite services could be utilized by other residential providers for similar reasons.

Respite Care Provider and Respite Care Giver: The person or persons who administers assistance in any form or fashion to the developmentally delayed persons.

Respite Care Recipient: The handicapped person or persons receiving the help of others in their day to day need for assistance.

Staff: All persons involved in the ministry to developmentally delayed persons.

Supervisors: The professional or para-professional who works with and guides the care activity of the developmentally delayed persons.

In some instances, names of persons have been altered to preserve anonymity.

APPENDIX 1

SOME OTHER FACILITIES NATIONWIDE

Portland State University *(see appendix II for resource listing)
Research and Training Center
Regional Research Institute for Human Services
P.O. Box 751
Portland, OR 97207-0751

Bay Area Family Services, Inc.
315 Henry Street
Valleho, CA 94591

DMR Region 5
Respite Care Program
104 S. Turnpike Road
Wallingford, CT 06492

Rest Assured Respite Program
United Cerebral Palsy of Tampa Bay
2215 E. Henry Avenue
Tampa, FL 33610

APPENDIX 2

RESEARCH AND TRAINING CENTER RESOURCE MATERIALS

- Annotated Bibliography, Parents of Emotionally Handicapped Children: Needs Resources, Relationships with Professionals. Covers relationships between professionals and parents, parent, problems and guidelines. $7.50 per copy.

- Annotated Bibliography, Youth in Transition: Resources for Program Developmental and Direct Service Intervention. Transition needs of adolescents: educational and vocational issues, programs and curriculum, search overviews, interpersonal issues, skills training. $6.00 per copy.

- Brothers and Sisters of Children with Disabilities: An Annotated Bibliography. Addresses the effects of children with disabilities on their brothers and sisters, relationships between children with disabilities and their siblings, services and education for family members. $5.00 per copy.

- Changing Roles, Changing Relationships: Parent-Professional Collaboration on Behalf of Children with Emotional Disabilities. The monograph examines barriers to collaboration, the elements of successful collaboration, strategies for parents and professionals to promote collaborative working relationships, checklist for collaboration, and suggested resources for further assistance. $4.50 per copy.

- Child Advocacy Annotated Bibliography. Includes selected articles, books, anthology entries and conference papers written since 1970, presented in a manner useful to readers who do not have an access to the cited sources. $9.00 per copy.

- Choices for Treatment: Methods, Models, and Programs of Intervention for Children with Emotional Disabilities and Their Families. An Annotated Bibliography. The literature written since 1980 on the range of therapeutic interventions used with children and adolescent with emotional disabilities is described. Examples of innovative strategies and programs are included. $6.50 per copy.

- Developing and Maintaining Mutual Aid Groups for Parents and Other Family Members: An Annotated Bibliography/topics addressed included the organization and development of parent support groups and self-help organizations, professional's roles in self-help groups, parent empowerment in a group leadership, and group advocacy. $7.50 per copy.

APPENDIX 3

VARIOUS FORMS TO FACILITATE DIFFERENT TYPES OF RESPITE CARE
(Our needs and Projections of Your Needs)

The following forms are developed for non-profit and "for profit" Respite Care. Both are needed. Hopefully these forms will alleviate burdensome administrative recordings of needed data. We have developed these forms with the hope our ministry might be multiplied and enlarged for greater Kingdom outreach. Feel free to select and duplicate what is seen as helpful in your situation.

PROFILE FOR RESPITE CARE CLIENT

Name_____

1. Do you reside in this County? _____

2. Age_____   Sex_____

3. Does your Care Recipient have a disability characterized as one of the

   following:

   3.1 _____mild mental retardation

   3.2 _____moderate mental retardation

   3.3 _____severe mental retardation

   3.4 _____epilepsy

   3.5 _____cerebral palsy/orthopedic

   3.6 _____autism

   3.7 _____emotional disturbances or other behavioral problems

   3.8 _____learning disability

   3.9 _____other physical or neurological impairments

   3.10 _____   non-verbal

   3.11 _____non-ambulatory

   3.12 _____visually impaired

   3.13 _____hearing impaired   ,

   3.14 _____medically at risk

   3.15 _____other, please be specific_____

4. My Care-Recipient currently resides:

4.1 _____ with parents

4.2 _____ with relatives

4.3 _____ alternative living program or other care home

4.4 _____ group home

4.5 _____ facility for intensive care/training

4.6 _____ nursing home

4.7 _____ institution (e.g. state hospital, state center, etc.)

4.8 _____ other please be specific

5. Please indicate your relationship to the Care Recipient

5.1 _____ parent

5.2 _____ guardian

5.3. _____ caretaker

5.4 _____ other, please specify_____

6. Check your age category please

6.1 _____ 15-19   6.5 _____ 46-55

6.2 _____ 20-25   6.6 _____ 56-65

6.3 _____ 26-35   6.7 _____ 66 and over

6.4 _____ 36-45

7. Please check the level of education you have completed:

<u>You</u> <u>Spouse</u>

7.1 ____ ____ grade school

7.2. ____ ____ some high school

7.3 ____ ____high school graduate

7.4 ____ ____some college

7.5 ____ ____college graduate

7.6 ____ ____vocational/tech/business school

7.7 ____ ____M.A. or equivalent

7.8 ____ ____beyond MA level

7.9 ____ ____other, be specific

8.   Marital Status   Ethnic Background

8.1____ married   8.1____ African American

8.2____ single   8.2 ____Anglo American

8.3____ divorced   8.3____ Hispanic American

8.4 ____widowed   8.4____ Native American

                     8.5____ Other, be specific

9.   Type of Employment

9.1____caretaker or guardian

9.2____parent or guardian

10. Indicate the ages of other children or dependents living in your home:

_____   _____   _____

_____   _____   _____

_____   _____   _____

11. Does your care recipient qualify for public assistance:

11.1 ____S.S.I.   11.4____ Social Security

11.2. ____Medicare   11.5____A.N.D.

11.3____Medicaid   11.6____ Other, be specific_____

12. Does anyone else in your household receive:

12.1____supplemental security income (SSI)

12.2 ____aid to families with dependent children

12.3____Social Security

12.4____other public assistance, be specific_____

REQUEST FOR RESPITE CARE

I.   Person or Agency requesting Service: (circle one)

      Social Worker   Foster Parent   Caretaker   Other

      Name and address of person requesting care:

      _____

      Name   Street   City   Zip Code   Phone

II.   Name of person to receive care:_____

      Address_____

      Age_____   Birthday_____   Disability_____

III.   Information about the person who will receive care:

      My care recipient's special needs are:

1. _____takes medication   6. _____feeds self

2. _____has seizures   7. _____dresses self

    _____uncontrolled   8. _____takes nap in

    _____controlled   _____afternoon

3. _____ can walk   _____morning

4. _____has some speech   9. _____is allergic (explain) _____

5. _____ is toilet trained

    _____fully   _____partially

    _____other

Brief description of individual's diagnosis, health & behavior

_____

Individual's special needs, likes, dislikes, favorite, pastimes, how he/she relates to strangers, others, etc.

_____

_____

Please give name of school, program or workshop attending:

_____

IV. Parents or Caretakers full name and address:

    Mother_____ Father_____

    Caretaker_____ Other_____

    Home:

    _____

    Street Address   City   Zip Code   Phone

    Marital Status: (circle one)   Single   Married   Divorced   Widowed

V. Caretaker's Employment (if any)

    Place of employment_____

    Address_____Phone_____

VI. Person to contact in case of emergency:

_____

_____

Full name   Relationship

_____

Address

_____

Home Phone Number_____Work Phone Number_____

VII. Information about other persons living at home:

Name   Age   Gender

1._____

2._____

3._____

4._____

VIII. Care preferences: I would prefer a care provider between the ages of:

___15 to 20   ___20 to 25   ___Older

I would prefer the care of my Care Recipient be done in:

_____my home   _____at church

_____care provider' home   _____other, please be specific

_____If my choice is not available, I give care provider permission to provide

other adequate care facility.

I will need Care Provider usually:

_____morning _____afternoon _____evening _____weekend

_____overnight

Transportation can be provided by:

_____myself _____the provider _____bus _____taxi

other_____

IX. Any other helpful information for the Care Provider:

_____

_____

_____

_____

PERTINENTS ABOUT OUR PROSPECTS

Name_____ birthdate_____ age_____

Address_____Zip code_____

Phone Number_____Email Address_____

Parents/Caretaker_____Date_____

Address_____Zip code_____

Telephone_____Email address_____

Eating

_____Must be fed junior or baby foods

_____Must be fed food from table

_____ (Does) (Does Not) hold bottle alone

_____Drinks from cup or glass (with) (without) assistance

_____Eats finger foods

_____Learning to use spoon - needs (much) (little) assistance

_____Uses spoon well alone

_____Completely self-sufficient at table

_____On special diet (Explain please)

_____Other (Explain please)

_____Has difficulty (swallowing) (chewing)

_____Uses food to manipulate caring persons (Explain person)

Mobility

IF INDIVIDUAL WEARS A PROSTHESIS OF ANY KIND, INDICATE ABILITIES TO USING IT (U), AND NOT ABLE TO USE (N).

_____Makes no attempt to move

_____ (Does) (Does not) (Tries to) roll over

_____Moves about on floor by (rolling) (scooting) (crawling) (other)

_____Pulls self up to standing position

_____Stands with assistance (hand, chair, etc.)

_____Stands alone

_____Takes at least 2 steps with assistance

_____Walks alone across room or further

_____Stumbles frequently, walks with furniture, doors, etc.

_____Walks alone with poor balance, does not fall

_____Walks (up) (down) stairs along or using bannister

_____Crawls or scoots (up) (down) stairs

_____Other (explain please)

Toileting

_____Toilet training not yet attempted

_____Currently working on toilet training

_____Care recipient indicates need to be assisted

_____Needs no assistance but must be reminded

_____Has accidents (daily) (weekly) (monthly or less) (in strange surroundings)

(when upset) or (excited)

_____Has accidents only at nights (indicate frequency above)

_____Completely self-sufficient in toileting

_____Uses toileting, bed wetting, etc. for attention

_____Other (please explain)_____

Communication

_____Smiles, laughs

_____Makes random vocalizations

_____Imitates sounds

_____Follows simple directions (come here, no, look, etc.)

_____Uses names of familiar objects or persona (ball, Daddy, etc.)

_____Talks in longer sentences

_____Relates experiences

_____Carries on conversation

_____Uses words but does not understand their meaning

_____Can speak, but refuses to do so

_____Indicates needs by crying, grunting, etc.

_____Indicates needs by pointing

_____Indicates needs by leading caregiver to door, cabinet, etc.

_____Speech is difficult for family to understand

_____Speech is difficult for strangers to understand.

_____Speech is understood by strangers after a few minutes

_____Speech is easily understood by strangers,

but therapy recommended (explain)

_____Speech quality is unimpaired

_____Other (Please explain)_____

Health Problems

_____None present

_____Hyperactive

_____Frequent upper respiratory infections.

_____Other respiratory ailments (asthma, pleurisy, etc.)

_____Impaired vision (please explain)

_____Impaired hearing (please explain)

_____Seizures (explain type, frequency, aura, if any; date of onset;

cause, if known, complications, even if seizures are now controlled)

_____Hydrocephalus (arrested?, how?)

_____Heart defect (please explain)

_____Color blindness

_____Drooling

_____Menstruation began at age

_____ (Does) (does not) care for self during period

_____Orthopedic difficulties (explain please - is surgery anticipated?

when? describe appliances requested

_____Give approximately date of past orthopedic treatment

_____Dental problems

_____Allergies (list please)

_____List all serious illnesses recently that might concern the developmentally

delayed persons caregivers

_____Any missing limbs

_____Metabolic disorders (please explain)

_____Neurological impairment (please explain)

List all medications currently given or prescribed, including doses and purposes.

_____

_____High tolerance to pain

_____Other (please explain)_____

Socialization

_____Reaches for familiar persons only

_____Enjoys being held and played with

_____Plays with or alongside others

_____Shies away from strangers

_____Plays cooperatively with others

_____Deliberately abuses or antagonizes others (explain

please)_____

_____Refuses to obey caretakers or others in authority

_____Prefers company of (older) (younger) persons or of adults

_____Prefers to be left alone

_____Becomes frustrated when_____

_____Handles frustration by_____

_____Responds to change in routine by_____

_____Responds to correction by_____

_____Describe interaction with household_____

Supervision Needed

_____Must be watched constantly

_____Plays (knowingly) (unknowingly) with dangerous objects if not watched

(be specific please)

_____Avoids sharp objects Avoids hot stoves and pans

_____Goes into street (or would if not watched) without safety precautions

_____Crosses streets safely after observing safety precautions

_____Not allowed to enter street alone (cannot safely)

_____Wanders away from home while awake

_____Wanders in sleep (within home) (away from home)

_____Takes supervision from others in authority

_____Can be left alone in house for 20 minutes

_____Can be trusted to watch younger children for 10 minutes

_____Behavior in public is (better than) (worse than) (same as) at home

_____ (Can) (cannot) be trusted not to take things from store shelves

without permission

_____ Takes things that do not belong to him/her (knowingly) (not knowingly)

that it does not belong to him/her

_____ Can be trusted to perform minor errands (mail letters, borrow an egg

from neighbors)

Personal Self-Help

_____ Fears bath

_____ Must be bathed

_____ Learning to bath self

_____ Bathes alone if water is run for him

_____ Runs water and bathes self, doing (good) (fair) (poor) job

_____ Tooth brushing not yet begun

_____ (Does) (does not) cooperate while teeth are brushed

_____ Learning to brush teeth

_____ Self-sufficient at tooth brushing (though reminders may be necessary)

_____ Recognizes "well groomed" and "sloppy" on (self) (others)

_____ Combs or brushes hair in (play) (grooming)

_____ (Shampoos) (sets) hair (alone) (with assistance)

_____ Does not help dress self

_____ Removes coat or dress alone if unfastened

_____ Puts on coat or dress (does) (does not) fasten it

_____Operates (zipper), (buttons), (snaps), (indicate which)

_____Ties shoestrings

_____Tells time to nearest (hour) (half hour) (quarter hour) (15 minutes)

_____Has the care recipient ever lived away from home? Yes_____ No_____

If so, please give dates and details._____

_____

Additional helpful comments:_____

_____

UP-DATE SHEET

I.   General Health (recent or prolonged illnesses):

_____

_____

_____

II.   Behaviors (anything out of the ordinary):

_____

_____

_____

III.   Habits (naptime, snacktime, schoolwork, mealtime):

_____

_____

_____

IV.   Medications:

_____

_____

_____

My care recipient takes:_____

It is to be administered:

How:_____

When:_____

V.   I/We can be reached in case of emergency at:_____

_____

The phone number:_____

The address is:_____

_____

VI.   My care recipient's physician is: _____

Phone: _____Email_____

Address:_____

VII.   In case of emergency and I cannot be reached, please call

1. Name_____

Relationship_____

Address_____

Phone_____Email_____

2. Name_____

Relationship_____

Address_____

Phone_____Email_____

VIII. General comments or observations:_____

_____

I have completed this form as the legal caretaker for Care Recipient

_____.

I have double checked all information and it is correct.

_____

Name of Parent/Caretaker

_____   _____

Signature of Parent/Caretaker   Date

AGREEMENT FOR RESPITE CARE

We/I (Mr., Mrs., Ms.) _____hereinafter

known as the caretaker, hereby known as respite care giver for the respite care of our

care recipient_____hereinafter known as respite care giver

for the respite care of our care recipient, age_____   said care to he rendered from the

respite care center at the_____.

This contract is effective from _____to_____

All services are free (gratis). Any expenses are to be paid by myself. We/I further agree

that any changes in this schedule be arranged by the respite care director.

We have carefully read and fully understand this contract and will abide by its

terms.

Respite Caretakers/parent

_____   _____
Mother   Date

_____   _____
Father   Date

_____   _____
Address   Phone

AUTHORIZATION FOR TREATMENT WITHOUT PRESENCE OF

PARENT OR CARETAKER

I_____, parent/caretaker of the Care

Recipient named below authorize the Church of God Respite Care Center for Developmentally Delayed Persons to act in my behalf in case of accident, injury or illness when immediate medical or surgical care is needed provided the above named individual makes a diligent effort first to notify me of the situation and obtain my preferences and consent. If efforts to notify me are unsuccessful, I authorize the above named individual or concern to take necessary action and give consent on my behalf as his judgment dictates.

Medical Responsibility: I further agree to assume financial responsibility in the event of accident or sickness of my care recipient while in the Respite Care ministry of the Savannah Church of God. If I cannot be reached, I hereby give permission to the above respite care provider to sign hospital operation permits for my care recipient for such operations or dental procedures as are considered necessary or desirable by medical judgment, including using anesthesia. I do prefer that the following physician(s) treat my care recipient:

Name   Address   Phone/Email

1.

2.

3.

Name of developmentally delayed person:_____

_____   _____
Witness   Signature of witness

_____   _____
Caregiver/Parent   Signature of Caregiver/Parent

ACCIDENT REPORT

Injured Person's Name:_____

Person's Name Filing Report:_____

Date:_____ Time:_____

Persons Present:_____

Please describe what occurred: _____

_____

_____

_____

Describe the physical condition of injured persons: (grogginess, imbalance, dilated eye

pupils, loss of consciousness, etc.)_____

_____

_____

_____

How long did any of the conditions last (please be specific)

_____

_____

_____

_____

Were the Respite Care Supervisor and Director notified? Yes____   No____

Date and Time _____

Were the Parent/Caretaker notified? Yes____ No____

Date and Time_____

First Aide Procedure(s), used and by whom? _____

_____

_____

Can anything be done to prevent the recurrence of this accident? _____

_____

_____

_____

_____

_____   _____   _____

Signature of Person Reporting   Caretaker/ Parent   Date

RESPITE CARE REQUISITION

_____   _____

Date care is needed   Respite Care Recipient & Caretaker

_____   _____

Hours Care is Needed   Caretaker's Phone Number

Date:_____Time:_____ Ethnic   Orientation:_____

Marital Status:_____

Respite Care Recipient's Name:_____

Address:_____Zip code_____

Home Phone_____Email_____

Work Phone_____

Request forms in:_____   Referred by:_____

Reason for request:_____   Care provided at:

Location_____

SPECIAL INFORMATION

Care Recipient's Name:_____

Age:_____   Birthdate:_____

Disability:_____

_____

_____

Staff Observation   (Give date and time of occasion)

_____

_____

_____

_____

_____

Any follow up suggested or done? Describe

_____

_____

_____

_____

RESPITE LOG FOR GENERAL PLACEMENT CARE
(Please make additional copies as needed)

Name of Caretaker:

Placement:

Date & Time

Brief Summary (to include caretakers location, respite care, and visit evaluation.)

Name of Caretaker:

Placement:

Date & Time

Brief Summary (to include caretakers location, respite care, and visit evaluation.)

Name of Caretaker:

Placement:

Date & Time

Brief Summary (to include caretakers location, respite care, and visit evaluation.)

CONSUMER CRITIQUE OF THE CHURCH'S D.D.P.

RESPITE CARE SERVICES

Please put the number which most accurately corresponds with your answer.

Unimportant 1   Somewhat Important 2   Important 3

Very Important 4   Urgent 5

I.   I use Respite Care because:

_____I need more time with my spouse

_____As a single caretaker, I need some rest and relaxation for myself

_____My developmentally disabled son/daughter/care recipient needs new

experiences and socialization

_____I need to spend more time with my non-disabled children

_____I need help with an occasional emergency

_____Other (please be specific_____

II.   Unexpected benefits received from using Respite Care:

_____Respite care is available when I need it

_____I am able to participate in social activities with my spouse

_____I feel comfortable leaving my developmentally delayed care

recipient assured of his/her care

_____Respite care can be done in my home as well as at the Care Center

_____My care recipient can be taken care of without difficult situation

evolving

94

III.   Personal Benefits continue to accrue:

_____Respite care has made a difference in my life

_____I can get counseling

_____I have made new friends plus finding an extended family I am

relieved of burdening my family for relief

Other (please be specific)_____

IV.   Before using the church's Respite Care, I seriously considered outside placement

for my developmentally delayed care recipient.

Yes_____   No_____

Since using the Respite Care of the church, I am able to better cope with our situation.

Yes_____   No_____

V.   I have found the Respite Caregiver to be:

Well prepared and capable

_____Genuinely interested in my care recipients well being

_____A person with good morals and a wholesome character

_____Easy to communicate with

_____Friendly

VI.   I have found the Church Respite Staff to be:

_____Knowledgeable and competent Cooperative

_____Genuinely interested in providing quality care

_____Available for counseling or to "just listen"

_____Helpful in crisis situations Easy to communicate with

VII.   Did you personally feel our Respite Care appropriate?

Yes_____   No_____

VIII. Would you use our Respite Care again? Yes_____   No_____

IX.   Would you recommend our Respite Care again? Yes_____ No_____

X.   Were you satisfied with our Respite Care? Yes_____   No_____

XI.   What difficulties, if any, did you or your care recipient encounter that you did not anticipate? (Please be specific)

_____

_____

_____

_____

XII.   Please state any other evaluations of this Respite Care Services.

_____

_____

_____

_____

We greatly appreciate you helping us by evaluating our Respite Care Service.

PROFILE FOR RESPITE CARE CLIENT

Name _____

1. In what city do you reside?_____

2. Age_____   Gender_____

3. Does your Care Recipient have a disability characterized as one of the

following:

     3.1   _____mild mental retardation.

     3.2   _____moderate mental retardation

     3.3   _____severe mental retardation

     3.4   _____epilepsy

     3.5   _____cerebral palsy/orthopedic

     3.6   _____autism

     3.7   _____emotional disturbance or other behavioral problems

     3.8   _____learning disability

     3.9   _____other physical or neurological impairments

     3.10   _____non-verbal

     3.11   _____non-ambulatory

     3.12   _____visually impaired

     3.13   _____hearing impaired

     3.14   _____medically at risk

     3.15   _____other, please be specific

4. My Care-Recipient currently resides:

4.1 _____with parents

4.2 _____with relatives

4.3 _____alternative living program or other care home

4.4 _____group home

4.5 _____facility for intensive care/training

4.6 _____nursing home

4.7 _____institution (e.g. state hospital, state center, etc.)

4.8 _____other, please be specific

5. Please indicate your relationship to the Care Recipient

5.1. _____Parent

5.2 _____Guardian

5.3 _____Care Taker

5.4 _____Other, be specific._____

6. Check your age category

6.1 _____15-19

6.2 _____20-25

6.3 _____26-35

6.5 _____46-55

6.6 _____56-65

6.7 _____66 and over

APPLICATION FOR RESPITE CAREGIVER

Mr./Mrs./Mrs._____
　　　　　First　　　　　　　Middle　　　　　　　Last

Spouse's name_____

Address_____
　　　Street　　　　　　　City　　　　State　　　Zip Code

Home Phone_____　　Birthdate_____

Children's Ages_____

Employed by_____

Position_____　　Business Phone_____

Liability Insurance (Homeowners or Renters Policy)

_____

Briefly state background, interests and/or experience working with handicapped

persons:_____

_____

_____

Availability for providing care:_____day _____hourly

_____evening　　　　_____night _____weekdays

_____weekends _____weekly _____monthly

Will care for persons: _____in own home _____in home of care recipient

_____no preference　　_____at church _____at outing

Education: (High School, College and Others)

Date Attended	Name & Address of School	Degree	Major

Employment (for last two years)

Dates Employed	Name & Address of Employer	Position Held

References (List 3 - other than relatives)

Name	Street	City	State	Zip Code

Do you speak any other languages?_____ Which ones?_____

How did you learn about the Respite Care Program?_____.

Date of Application_____ Signature_____

CHAIR/DIRECTORS INTERVIEW FORM

A.   Name_____

      Address_____

      Telephone Number_____Email_____

      Liability Insurance Church Activity Policy_____

      _____

B. Family Composition:

	Age	Gender
Parents		
Children		
Other		
Pets		
Dog(s)		
Cat(s)		
Other		

C. Health: General Health of Caregiving Members

_____

_____

_____

_____

List here any conditions which you are aware of that would restrict or limit the on-going care offered by the caregivers, for example, cardiac, frequent cold, physical handicaps, hypertension, etc.

Caregiver   Limitations

_____

_____

_____

_____

Check for any overt or admitted health problems, ask prospective Respite Caregivers to discuss their plans to offer Respite care with their physicians and to obtain his/her approval before committing themselves to this ministry. (If there is any need to obtain a certificate of good health from their physicians-please do so).

Emotional Health: What is the overall feel of the staff about working together?

_____

_____

_____

How do the caregiving members use their leisure time?_____

_____

What are their fun or pleasure activities?_____

_____

Ask the Respite Caregivers how the addition of handicapped persons to the program will affect the preceding activities?

_____

_____

_____

According to your observation, what is your church's motivation for offering Respite Care to Developmentally Delayed Persons?

_____

_____

_____

Enumerate some types of handicaps your Respite Caregivers feel secure about handling?

_____

_____

_____

What types of handicaps do the Respite Caregivers feel inadequate to handle?

_____

_____

_____

Do you feel confident in your abilities to handle your staff under ordinary circumstances? _____ In emergency?_____

D.   References:

Please supply identities, addresses and phone numbers of two persons (not relatives) who know the Respite Caregivers.

_____

_____

E.   Care Provider's Availability:

Hourly - Day

     Evenings

How often_____   Every week_____   Other_____

F.   Further Comments:

_____   _____

Interviewer   Date

STAFF REFERENCE FORM 1

Applicant's Name:

Any Particulars:

1. How long have you known the applicant? In what capacity? Explain.

   _____

   _____

2. Do you have reasons to question the applicant's moral standards? If so, please answer.

   _____

   _____

3. In your opinion, is the applicant emotionally stable?

   _____

   _____

4. What are your observations regarding the applicant's reliability and dependability?

   _____

   _____

5. To your knowledge, do children have a positive response to the applicant?

   _____

   _____

6. Do you know of any reasons whereby the applicant is unsuited for child or D.D.P. care? Situationally, home, outings at church, etc.?

_____

_____

7. From your personal observation, what helpful comments can you make affirmative or negative?

_____

_____

All information tendered will be held in confidence.

Reference's Name (Please Print) _____

Signature of Reference _____

Address_____

Phone_____Email_____

RESPITE CAREGIVER'S EVALUATION OF THE CHURCH'S D.D.P.

CARE SERVICE

Please fill in the blank with the number which most accurately fits your answer.

Unimportant l;   Somewhat Important 2;   Important 3;   Very Important 4;

Urgent 5

1.   I provide Respite Care because:

_____I am genuinely interested in assisting families with a Developmentally

Delayed member

_____I am a caretaker of a developmentally disabled child/adult

_____I want to use my free time constructively

_____I feel the burden of this ministry Other (please state reason)

2.   I was recruited to be a Respite Caregiver through:

_____Church bulletin

_____Respite Care Staff Presentation

_____The Pastor

_____Telephone Ministry

_____ Newspaper article

_____A friend

_____Church member

_____Other, please specify_____

Please evaluate the following by using Poor 1; Fair 2; Average 3; Good 4; Excellent 5

3.   My training by the Respite Care Staff was: _____

4.   I have found the Church's D.D.P. Respite Care Staff to be:

     _____Knowledgeable and competent Cooperative

     _____Genuinely interested in providing quality care

     _____Available when I need them

     _____Helpful in problem situations

     _____Easy to communicate with

5.   The Caregiver's panel was: _____

6.   Do you feel you are sufficiently informed regarding the special needs of your care recipient? Yes_____   No_____

If no, what additional information would you have preferred? (Please be specific)

7.   Did you encounter unforeseen difficulties? (Please be specific)

8.   After your involvement, would you recommend Respite Care to Developmentally Delayed Persons? Yes_____   No_____

9.   Do you think a fee should be charged? Yes _____   No_____

10.   From your observation point, how do you think the service can be improved by the Staff? (Please be specific)

Your help in evaluating our service is greatly appreciated. Thank you kindly.

BIBLIOGRAPHY

Appollini, A. H. and G. Triest, "Respite Services in California: Status and Recommendations for Improvements". Mental Retardation 21, 1983: n.p. 235-243

Association for Retarded Citizens. Characteristics of Respite Care Programs. Arlington, TX, 1982: n.p.

Bogardus, LaDonna. Christian Education for Retarded Persons. Nashville, New York: Abington Press, n.d.

Carlson, Bernice Wells, and David R. Gingeland. Play Activities for the Retarded. Nashville, TN: Abington Press, 1961.

Cox, Carole B. Community Care for an Aging Society: Issues, Policies, and Services. New York, NY: Springer Publishing Company, Inc. 2005.

Darling, R.B. Family Against Society: A Study of Reactions to Children With Birth Defects. - California Sage Publications, 1979.

Dongan, Teirell, Lyn Isbell and Pat Vyas. We Have Been There. Abington Press, 1983.

Dunlap, W.R. "How Do Parents of Handicapped Children View Their Needs?" Journal of the Division of Early Childhood 1. 1969: n.p. 1-10

Eriksson, Hans Goran and Torill Tjelfaat , Residential Care: Horizons for the New Century, Burlington, VT : Ashgate Publishing Company, 2004

Finnice Nancie R. Handling the Young Cerebral Palsied Child at Home. New York • E.P. Dutton, n.d.

Foote, Christopher and Christine Stanners, Integrating Care for Older People: New Care for Old – A Systems Approach Philadelphia, PA: Jessica Kinsley Publisher Ltd, 2002

Kirk, Samuel A. Early Education of the Mentally Retarded. Urbanna, IL: University Press, 1958.

Knapp, Martin and David challis, Long-Term Care: Matching Resources and Needs, Burlington, VT: Ashgate Publishing Company, 2004

Knight, Abigail, <u>A Straightforward Guide to Caring for a Disabled Child</u>.
 Straightforward Publishing Limited. 2004

Laverty, Helen and Mary Reet, <u>Planning Care for children in Respite Settings</u>
 Philadelphia, PA: Jessica Kinsley Publisher Ltd, 2001

Montgomery, Rhonda J. V., PhD. <u>A New Look at community-Based Respite Programs:
 Utilization, satisfaction, and Development, Volume 21,</u> New York, NY: The
 Haworth Press, Inc. 2002

Portland State University. <u>Research and Training Center on Family Support and
 Children's Mental Health.</u> Green Bay, WI: The Texas Respite Resource
Network, n.d.

Purdey, Jane. <u>Respite Care: A Guide For Parents Manual.</u> Washington: CSR, Inc., n.d.

The author, Dr. Isaac Croom Turner, is available for interviews and/or speaking engagements. Please contact him at 313.598.9708.

To order additional copies of the book, please send a check or money order in the amount of $16.95 per book, plus $3.00 for shipping and handling to:

Dr. Issac C. Turner
Reconciliation-Respite Ministries
Box 302
Troy, MI 48099-0302

Make checks payable to: Isaac C. Turner

Printed in the United States
91547LV00002B/247-330/A

9 780979 697845